LEICESTERSHIRE
COUNTY COUNCIL
LIBRARIES AND
INFORMATION SERVICE

Charges are payable on books overdue at public libraries. This book
is due for return by the last date shown but if not required by
another reader may be renewed — ask at the library, telephone
or write quoting the last date and the details shown above.     G3

# Proteins

by Jane Inglis

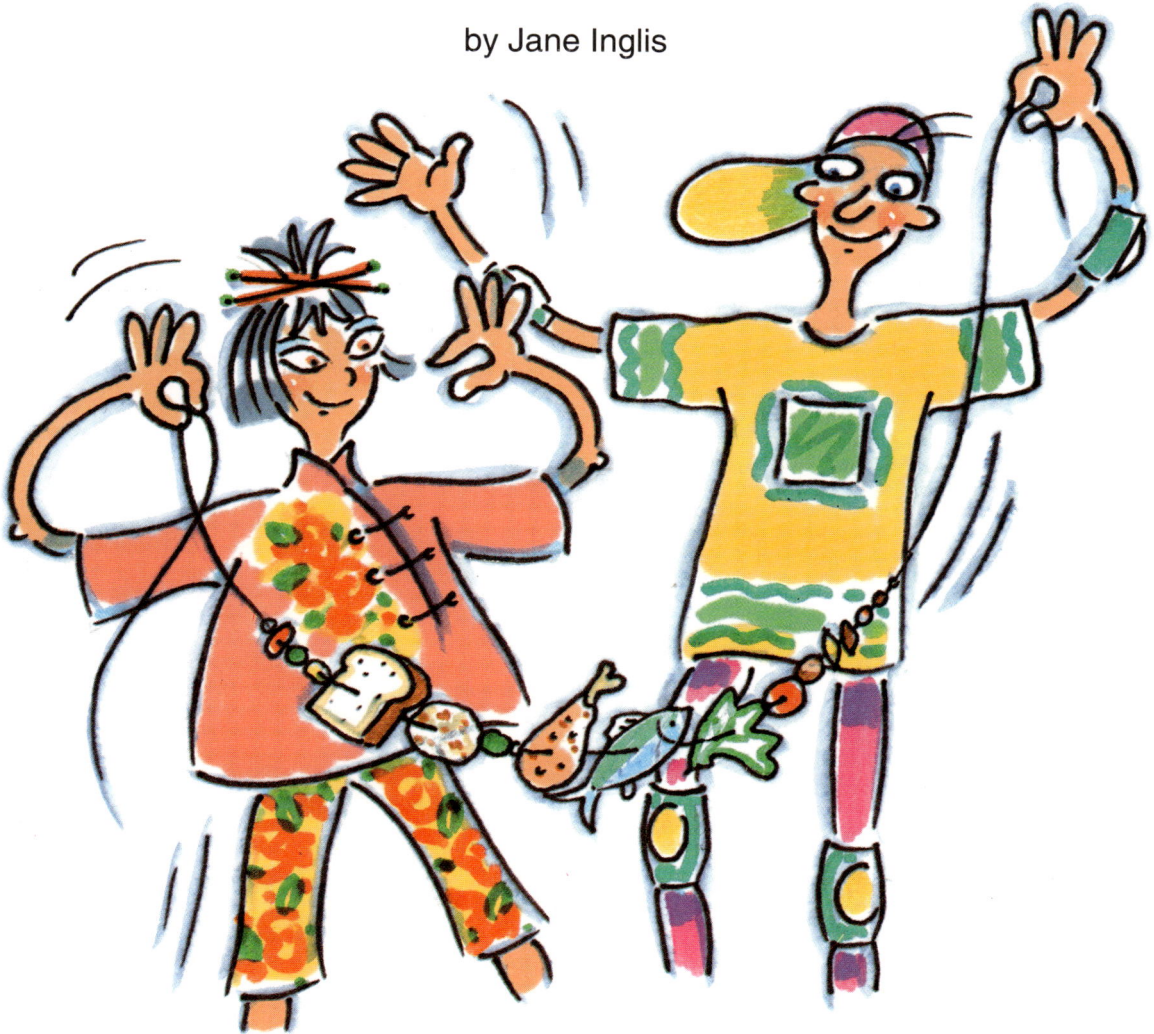

Wayland

Additives
Vitamins
Fibre
Sugar
Fats
Proteins

Words printed in **bold** can be found in the glossary on page 30.

First published in 1992 by Wayland (Publishers) Ltd.
61 Western Road, Hove, East Sussex, BN3 1JD

**British Library Cataloguing in Publication Data**

Inglis, Jane
  Proteins. – (Food Facts)
  I. Title II. Series
  613.2

  ISBN 07502 0514 8

*Series Editor:* Kathryn Smith
*Designer:* Helen White
*Artwork:* John Yates
*Cartoons:* Maureen Jackson

Typesetting by White Design
Printed and bound in Belgium by Casterman S.A.

# Contents

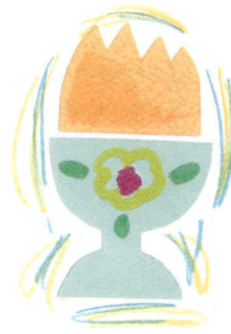

# Protein

names of some of them. They are: protein, fat, carbohydrates, vitamins and minerals. Our bodies need all of them to do different jobs.

This book is about one of the most important nutrients; protein. Every human being needs the right amount of protein to grow up strong and healthy. This book will tell you how much protein you need and how to get it from your food. It also looks at the problem of feeding all the hungry people in the world today, and the even bigger problem of how to grow enough protein for a much greater number of people, as the **population** of the world keeps on growing.

**What is protein?**

The word protein tells us how important it is. It comes from a Greek word meaning prime or basic. All the nutrients are important, but protein is the most basic of all because our bodies could not grow without it. Although we usually talk about protein, there are actually lots of kinds of protein.

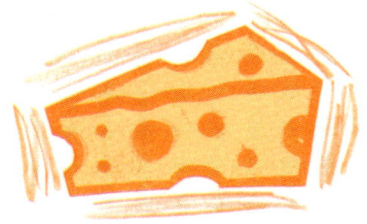

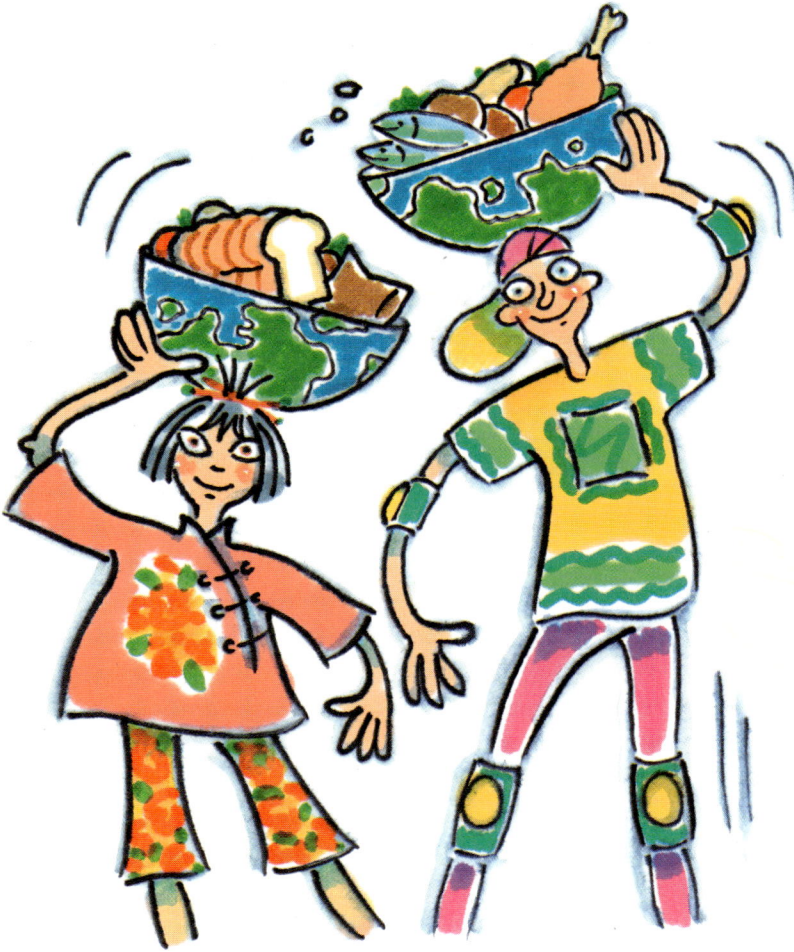

*OPPOSITE* Every human being needs the right amount of protein to grow up healthy. But every human being is different, so the right amount of protein is different for each of us.

Everyone knows that people need food to stay alive. When we are young we need it to grow too. There are lots of different, useful things in food. They are called **nutrients**, and there are five main kinds of nutrient needed by our bodies. You probably know the

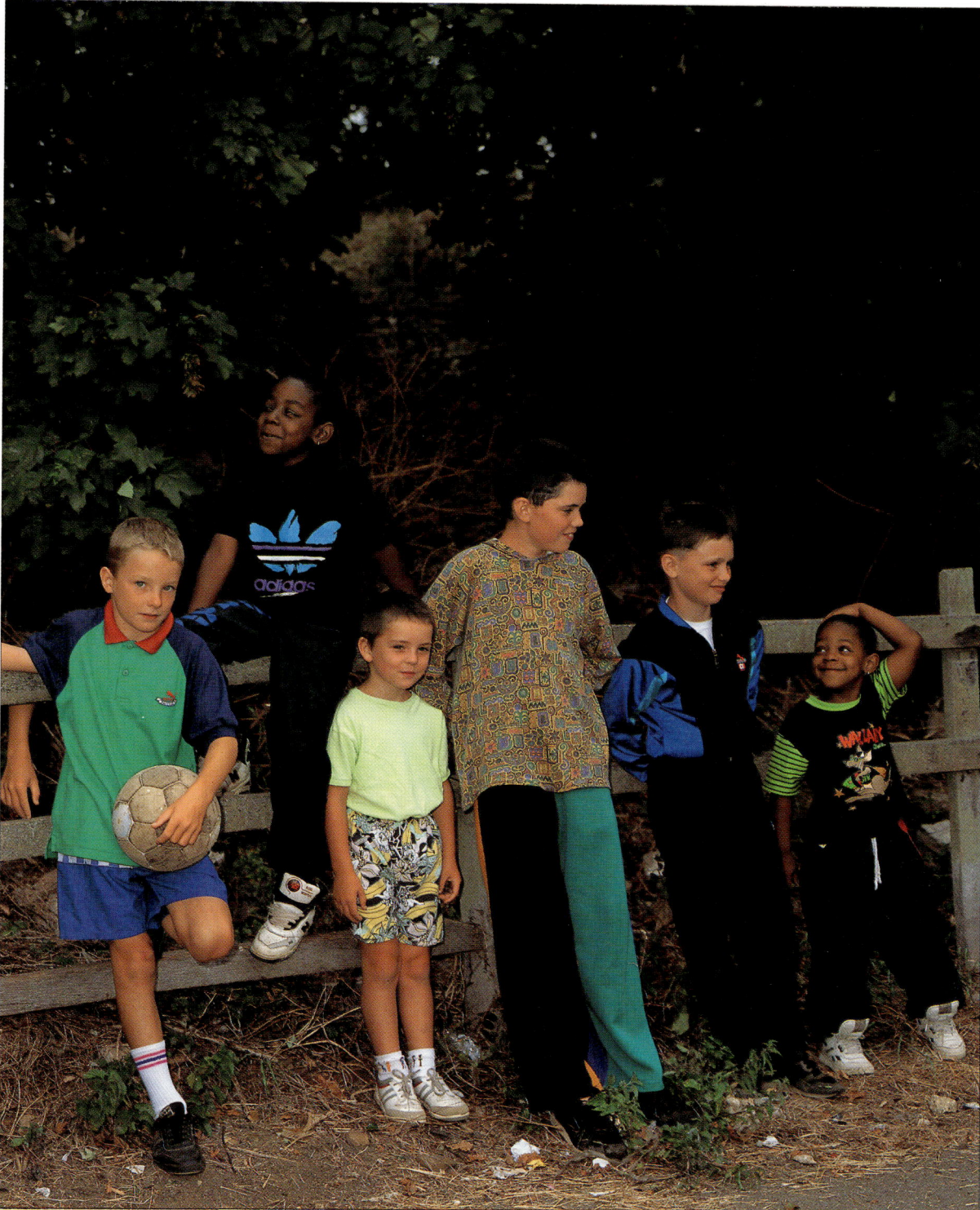

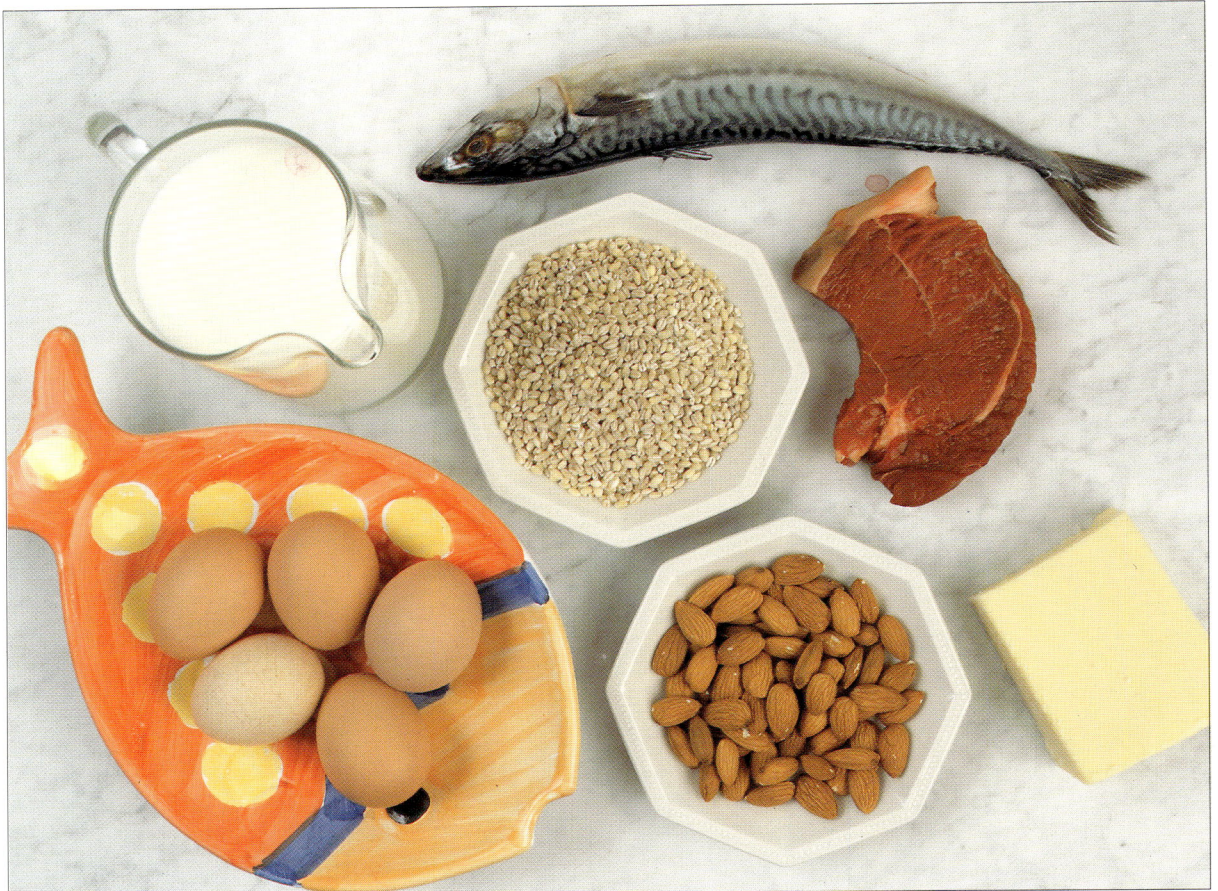

Our bodies need many of these different kinds of protein. Their job is to build the body and to keep it healthy.

Every living thing is made up of millions of tiny parts called **cells**, and every cell has proteins in it. Even when we are grown up, our cells are changing all the time and need protein. But children need it even more because their bodies are making new cells as they grow.

You can see some of the new cells your body has made if you look at your hair and your nails. These keep growing all the time, and your body uses the protein from your food to make new nails and new hair. If your hair and nails are healthy you can be sure you are getting enough protein.

About 20 per cent of the weight of your body is protein. It's found not only in your hair and nails, but also in your skin, your muscles and even in your bones. Different kinds of protein keep your blood healthy, help the body to use the food you eat, and fight off illness.

Some of the nutrients our bodies get from food can be stored, so that we don't need to eat food containing them every day. But we do need a new supply of protein every day.

*RIGHT* Your body uses some of the protein from your food to make new hair. If your hair is shiny and healthy, you can be sure you are getting enough protein.

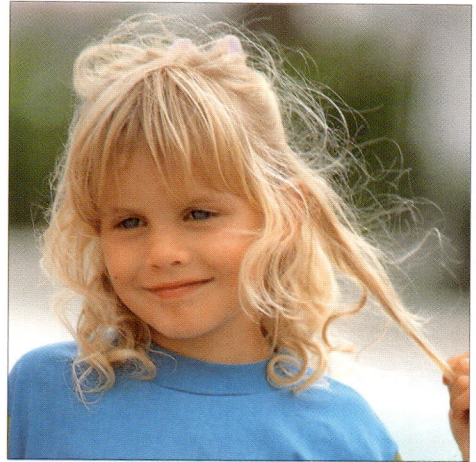

## Science corner

How much of your body weight is protein?
To find out, weigh yourself on a set of scales. If you are wearing clothes, take 1 kg off your weight. To work out roughly the weight of protein in your body, divide your body weight by five.

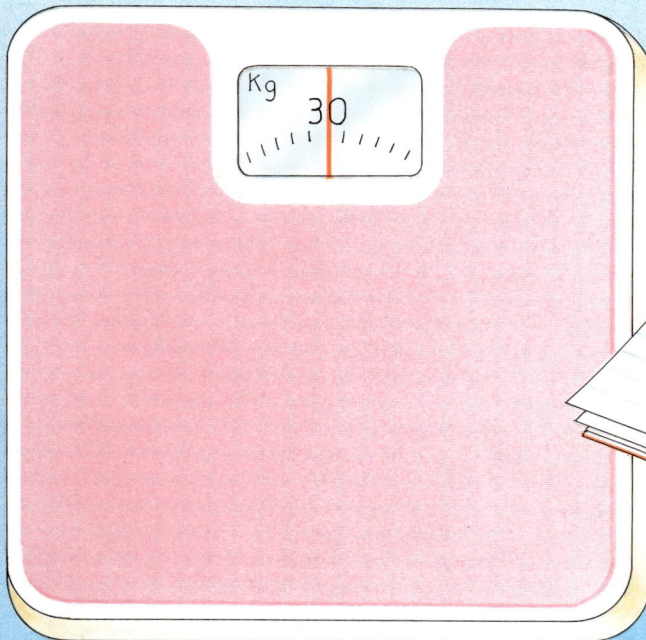

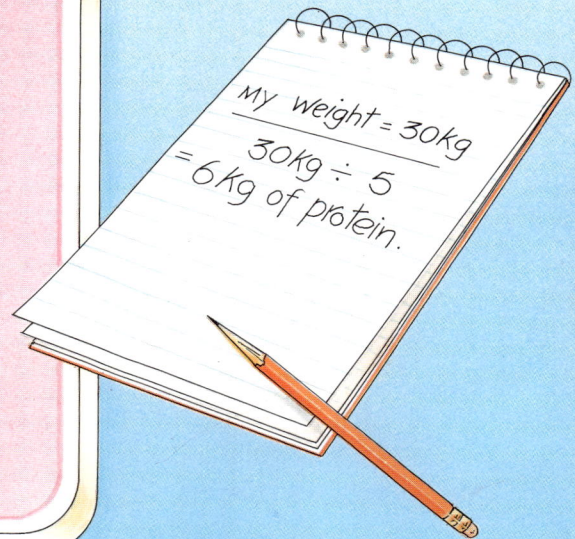

Kg
30

My weight = 30kg

30kg ÷ 5
= 6kg of protein.

# What are proteins made of?

All the different kinds of protein have been studied for years by **experts**, and we now know quite a lot (though not everything) about what they are made of. The building blocks that make up proteins are called **amino acids**. At least twenty-two different amino acids are now known, and these can be arranged in lots of ways to make up the different kinds of protein.

*BELOW* These nuts contain just some of the proteins we need to keep our bodies fit and healthy. We could not get all our proteins from nuts; we need other proteins too, which are found in different types of food.

To get an idea of how many different kinds of protein can be made from these amino acids, just think of the twenty-six letters of the alphabet. All the words in the English language are made up of these letters, arranged in different ways. Or think of twenty-two different kinds of beads, which could be strung together to make lots of different necklaces. All the proteins that do

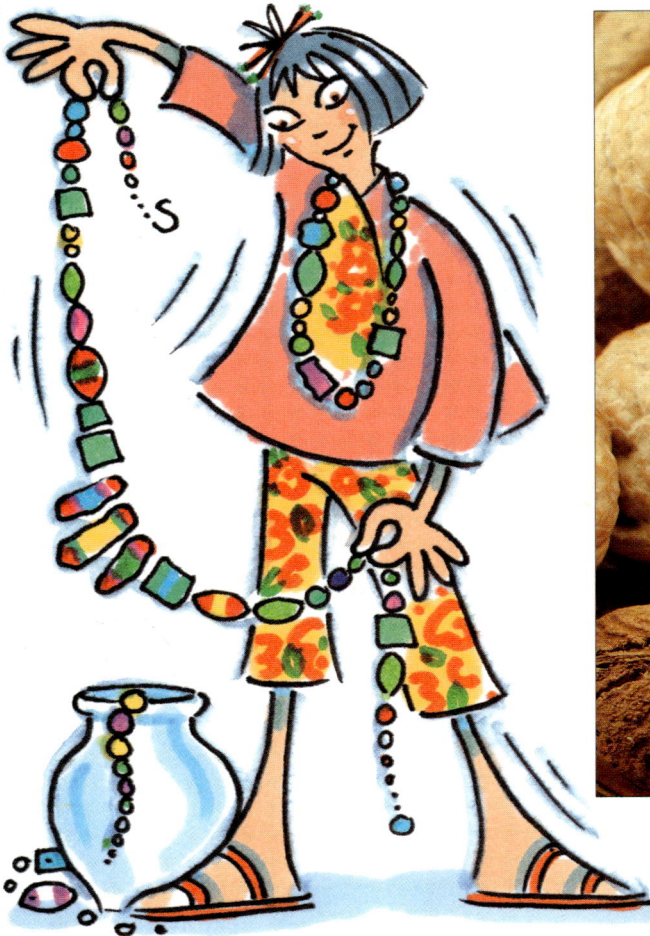

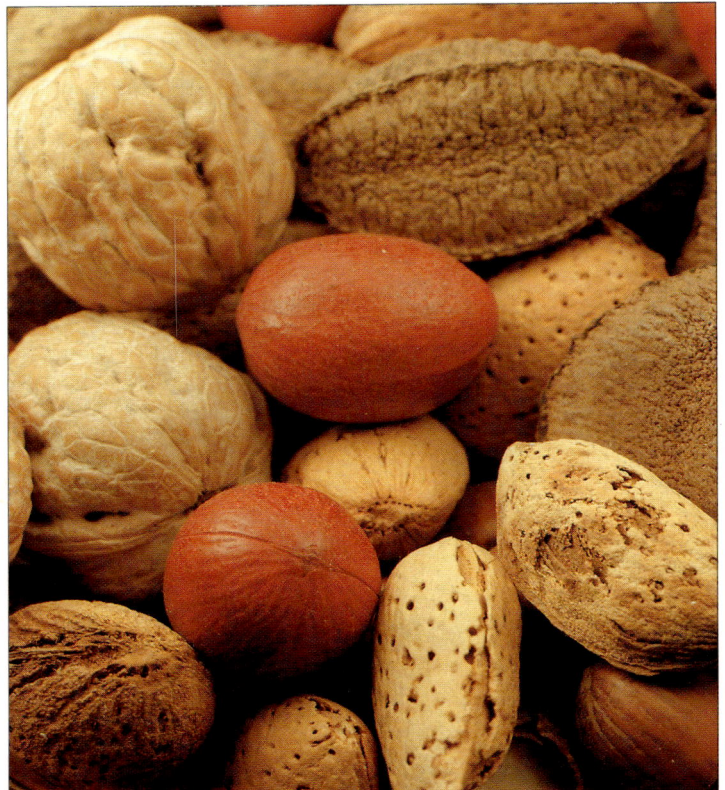

all the different jobs needed by our bodies are made up of these amino acids, arranged in different ways like beads on a string or letters in words.

Our bodies can make most of these amino acids for themselves, but eight of them cannot be made by the body. They must come from food, ready-made for our bodies to use. They are essential, something we must have, so they are sometimes called essential amino acids (EAAs). Children need an extra two amino acids while they are growing.

The story of protein is really the story of how we get these essential amino acids. It is not a simple story, and experts have studied it for years without agreeing about all the details. One reason for this is that people are not all exactly alike. Different people need different amounts of protein, and the same person may need a different amount at different times. All over the world people eat very different kinds of food and get their protein in different ways.

It's not easy to study such a huge subject, but it is important to know about what we eat, if we want to stay healthy.

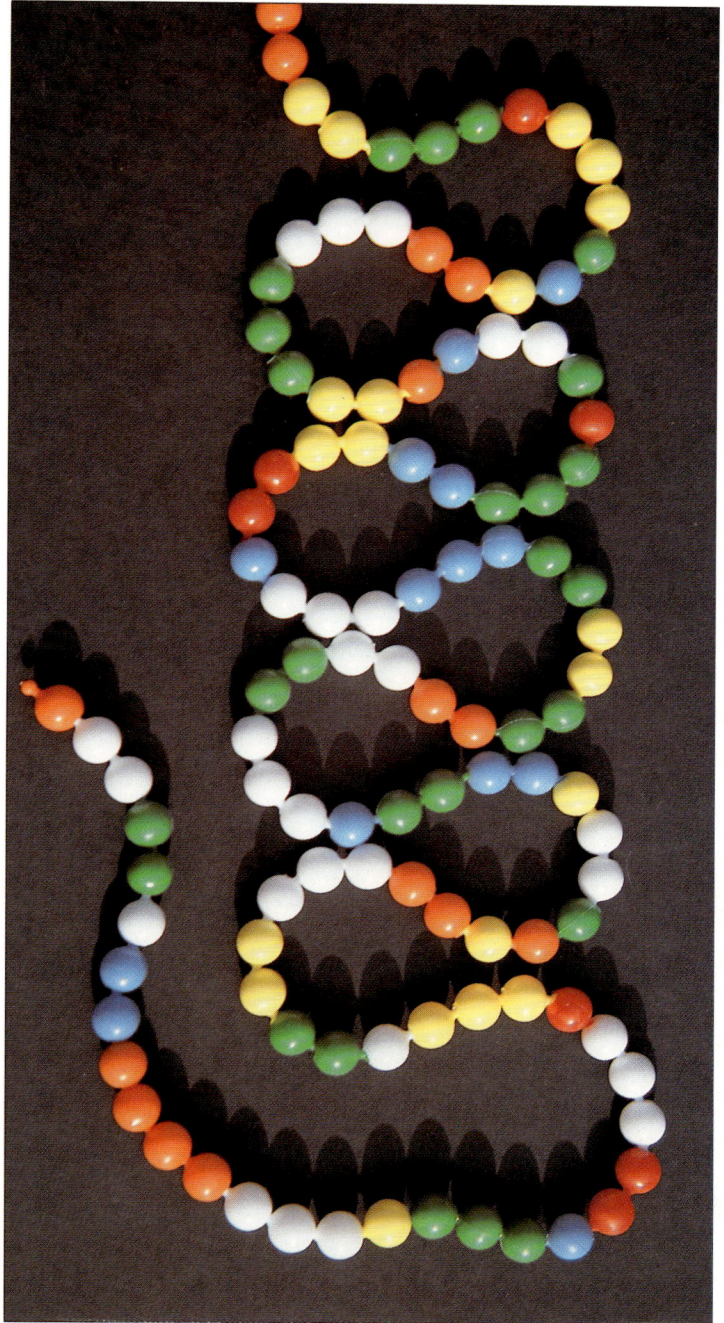

*ABOVE* These beads are like a protein; they are the amino acids, strung together in a pattern, to make one type of protein.

**Science corner**

This experiment is easier if you can do it with a big group of children; twenty-two is ideal! Everyone decides on a shape and colour (for example, red square, blue triangle, yellow star and green circle). No two should be the same. Draw, colour in and cut out at least ten copies of your shape. All the shapes are then mixed up. Each child should take ten shapes from the pile. Now you can arrange your shapes in rows, to get some idea of the variety of proteins that can be built up from twenty-two amino acids. If you thread them on a string you will have a model of part of a protein.

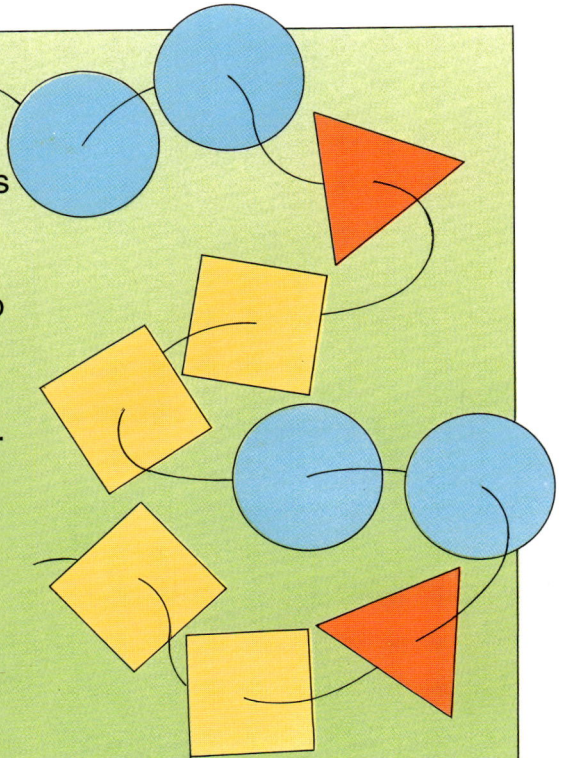

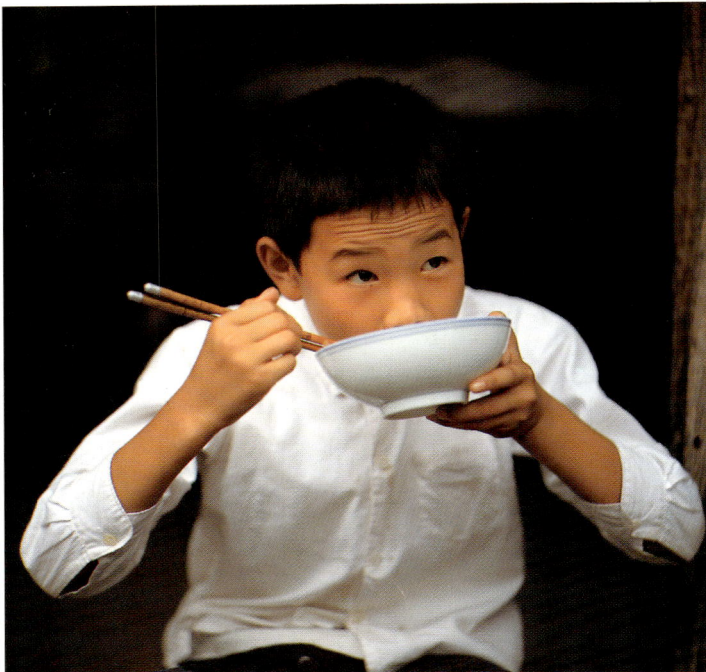

We also need to think about how we can change the way we eat. We might want to do this to be more healthy. We might want to eat in a way that is better for our planet, or in a way that helps to share out the food grown all over the world more fairly. You probably know a grown-up who wants to change the way they eat so that they lose weight! There are lots of reasons for finding out as much as we can about the food we eat. The more we know, the easier it will be to decide what we want to eat.

# A bunch of EAAs

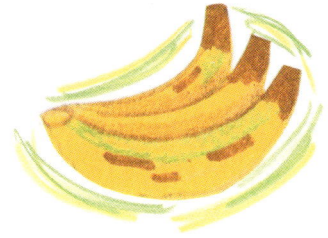

Your body needs to get the eight (or ten, if you are a growing child) essential amino acids in the right amounts, in order to remain healthy. Not all proteins in food give us exactly the right amounts of these EAAs. If there is too little of one, the body cannot use all of the others. We have to get those eight EAAs in the right pattern in order to be able to use them.

To help you to understand this, imagine a builder using an **architect's** design to build a house. The house must have so many bricks in the walls, so many tiles on the roof, so many doors and windows. If he or she had twice the right number of bricks and half the number of tiles, the house could not be built properly. Half the roof would be missing, the extra bricks would be no use, and the doors and windows would be wasted.

OPPOSITE In China people get their protein from a diet of rice, mixed with vegetables, fish or meat.

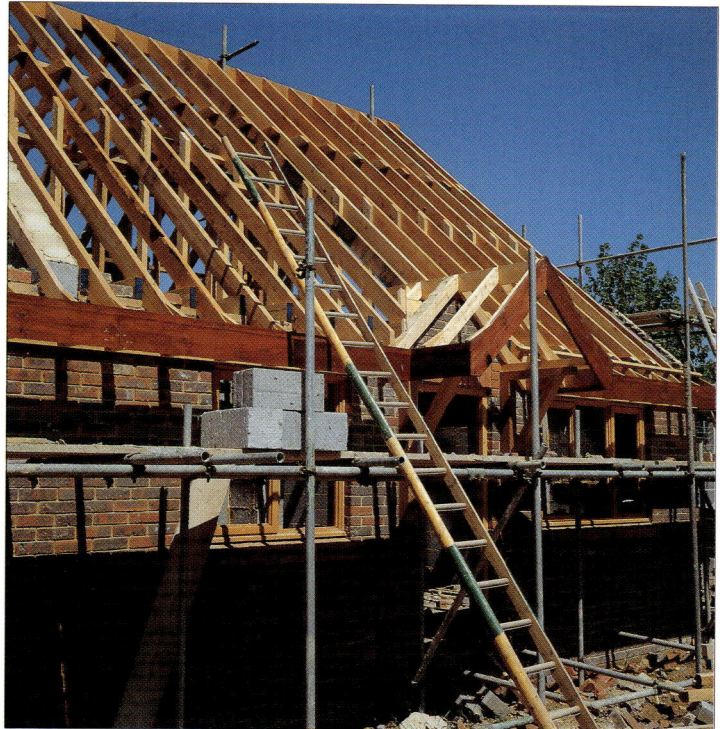

ABOVE A builder needs the right sort and amount of materials to build a house. In the same way, we need exactly the right sort and amount of amino acids to build a strong, healthy body.

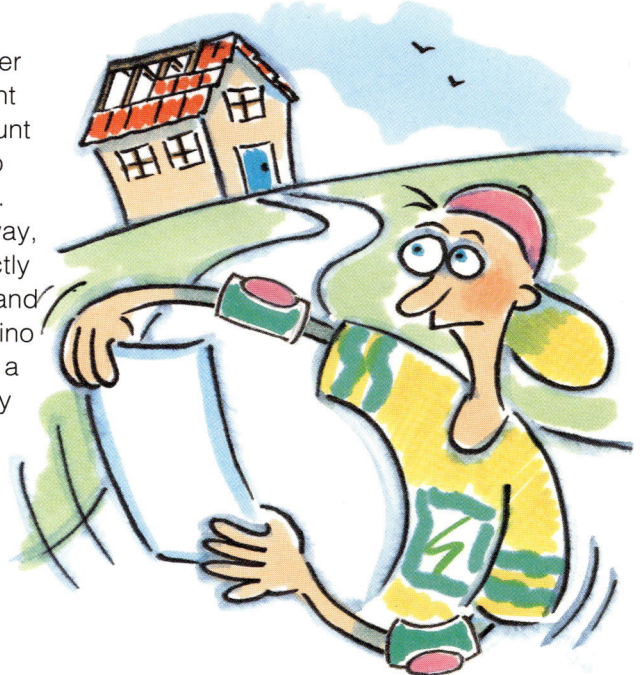

11

## Science corner

To illustrate what happens when we do not get the right mix of essential amino acids, you can do this quick experiment. Take one of the strings of shapes you made from the last science corner. Imagine it is the pattern for the protein needed by the human body. Now add on any number of extra shapes to the string. The extra ones will be wasted by the body because they do not fit the pattern.

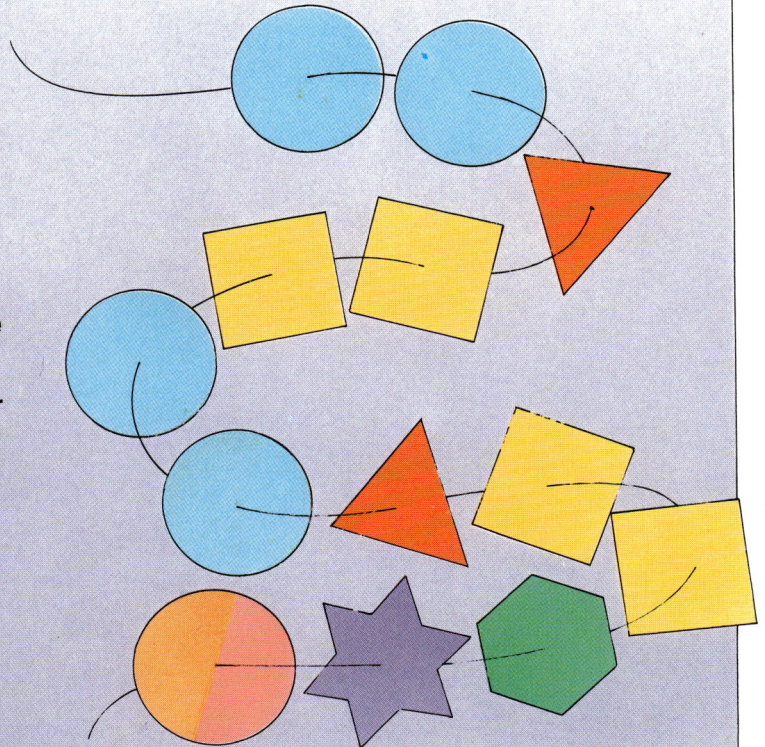

When our bodies take protein from the food we eat, they need to get the EAAs in the right amounts, like the builder who needs ten doors, sixteen windows and 15,000

*LEFT* Eggs contain the best mixture of essential amino-acids (EAAs) for our needs.

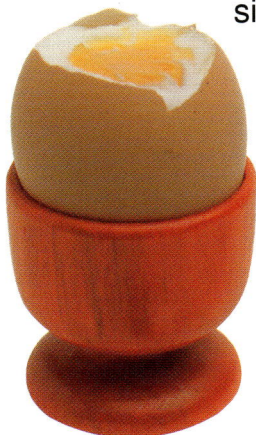

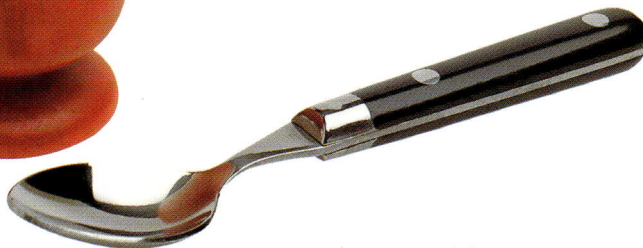

bricks if he or she is to be able to build the house the right shape and size.

Of all the foods that give us protein, eggs have the best mixture of EAAs for our needs. All the protein we get from eggs can be used by our bodies because there is the right amount of each EAA. This does not mean that we could or should rely on eggs as our only way of getting protein! It would be very boring to eat such a lot of eggs, and bad for our health too. Like all foods, eggs contain a mixture of lots of nutrients, not just protein. They are high in fat, so that one egg a day is probably too many.

In any case, there is no need to stick to one kind of food just because the pattern of EAAs is right. We can put different foods together so that the mixture contains the right amount of all the EAAs.

*BELOW* We need different amounts of protein at different times in our lives. Young children need lots of protein to give them energy and to make new cells, in order to grow.

This means that we can get all the protein we need using lots of different kinds of food. Long before experts worked it all out, people all over the world had found ways of eating that used a mixture of foods to get good quality protein.

## How much protein do we need?

This question has been answered in many different ways by experts. We do need different amounts of protein at different times in our lives.

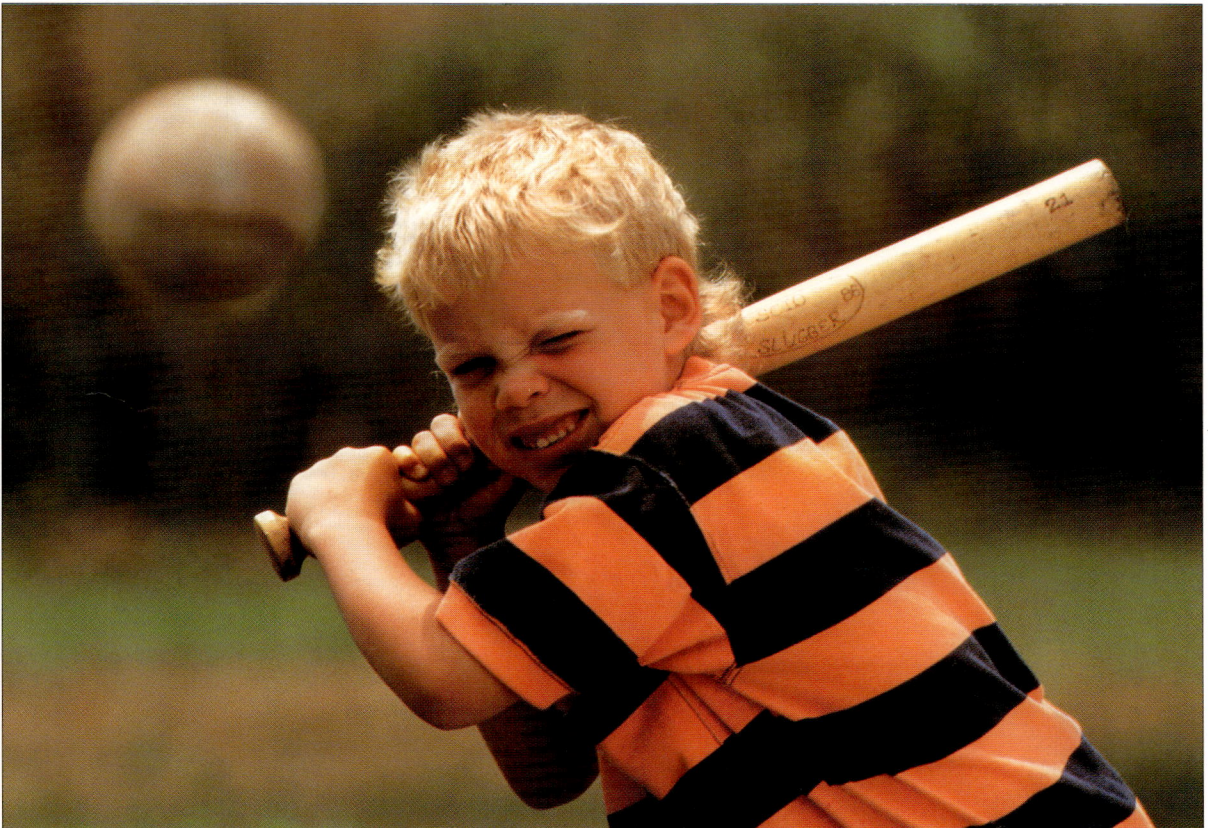

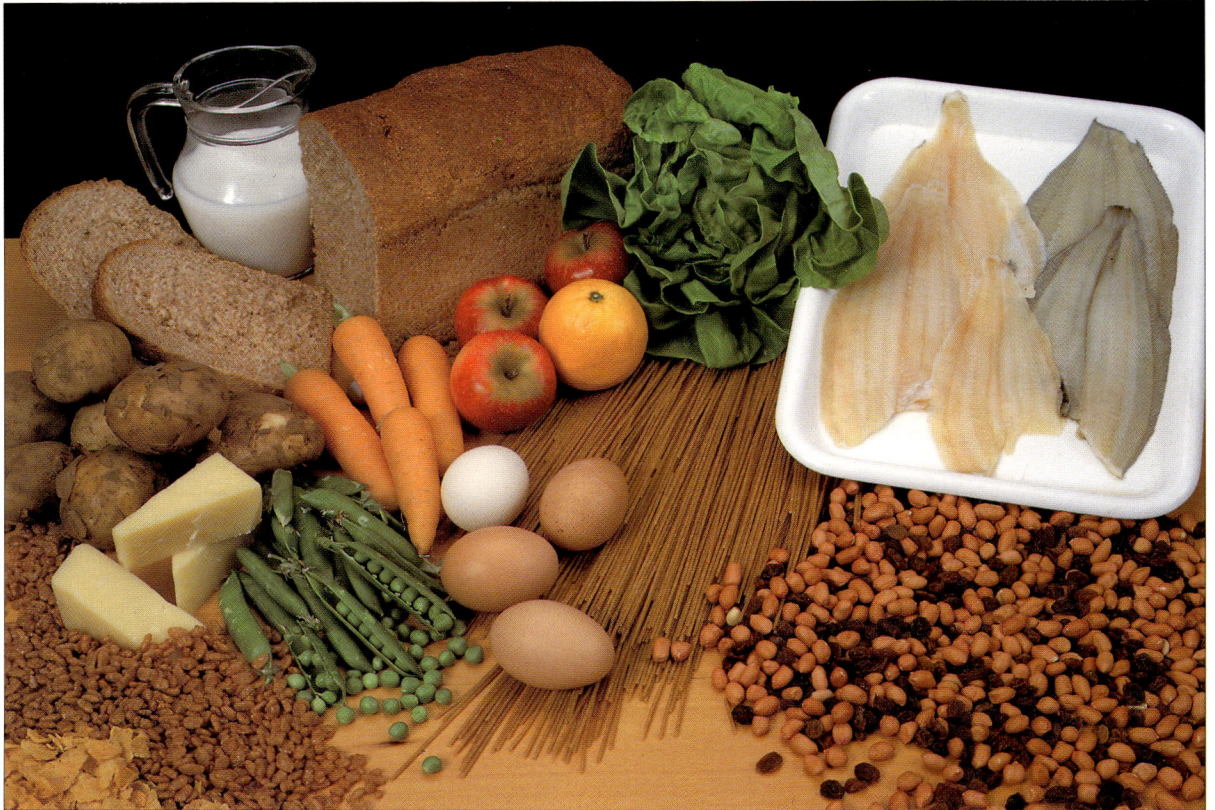

*ABOVE* These foods contain the five most important nutrients; protein, vitamins and minerals, carbohydrates, fats and fibre. If we eat a diet which contains all five of these nutrients in the correct amount, our bodies have a good chance of staying healthy.

Children need lots because they are growing. Teenagers need plenty as they shoot up. Pregnant women need enough to feed the growing baby, and nursing mothers need lots of protein to make milk. We all need more when we're ill or under stress. But the old idea that very large amounts of protein were needed by athletes and other people who lead very active lives is now out of fashion. In fact some experts think that it is bad for us to have too much protein.

## Protein overload?

Once the body has taken all the protein it needs from the food we eat to build new cells and keep healthy, it can 'burn up' any extra protein to get energy. But energy also comes from the carbohydrates we eat and from fats. These foods are cheaper, so it is wasteful to use protein for energy. It may also be hard on the body. Some experts think that it's a strain to **convert** a great deal of protein from food into energy. It may even damage the body.

Eating very large amounts of protein helps quick growth early in life, but people who go on eating like this all their lives may show signs of old age much too soon, and may live for a shorter time. Some studies show that cancer and other killer diseases are more common in people who eat very large quantities of protein. Table 1 shows the amount of protein needed by people of different ages.

To use this table, you need to understand the idea of an average. If you have a group of six children between seven and ten years old, they will all weigh different amounts. To find their average weight, you add up all six different weights, and divide by six. The answer is the average weight for that group of children.

Tables like this one, that tell you how much you need of this or that, always use the idea of an average. If you are much bigger or much smaller than most children your age, you will need a little more or less than the amount of protein given in the last column. It does not matter at all if you are very different. People will always be different in all kinds of ways. An average does *not* tell you what you should be. It is just useful to tell you roughly how much of something you might need.

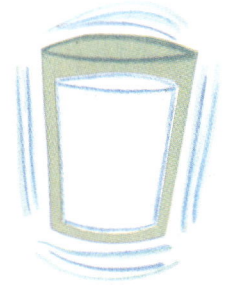

## Table 1

### Recommended daily amounts of protein.

|  | Average height (cm) | Average weight (kg) | Protein (gm) |
|---|---|---|---|
| Children 4-6 years | 112 cm | 20 kg | 30 g |
| Children 7-10 years | 132 cm | 28 kg | 34 g |
| Children 11-14 years | 157 cm | 45 kg | 45 g |
| Teenager (male) 15-18 | 176 cm | 66 kg | 56 g |
| Teenager (female) 15-18 | 163 cm | 55 kg | 46 g |
| Adult male | 177 cm | 70 kg | 56 g |
| Adult female | 163 cm | 55 kg | 46 g |

## Science corner

Get into small groups and work out the average weight and height of the group.

1. Weigh and measure the height of everyone in the group, carefully noting down your results.
2. To work out the average weight of the group, add together the weights of everyone in the group, and then divide your answer by the number of people in the group. The answer will be the average weight of the group.
3. To work out the average height of the group, follow the same method, using the height measurements you noted down.

Compare your results with the figures in the table on page 15. Decide how much protein each person needs.

| Name | Height | Weight | |
|------|--------|--------|---|
| 1. John | 128 cm | 28 kg | Average height = |
| 2. Sue | 132 cm | 30 kg | $4\overline{)515} = 128 \cdot 75$ cm |
| 3. Samara | 130 cm | 26 kg | Average weight = |
| 4. Mita | 125 cm | 29 kg | $4\overline{)113} = 28 \cdot 25$ kg |
| total: | 515 cm | 113 kg | |

# Which foods contain protein?

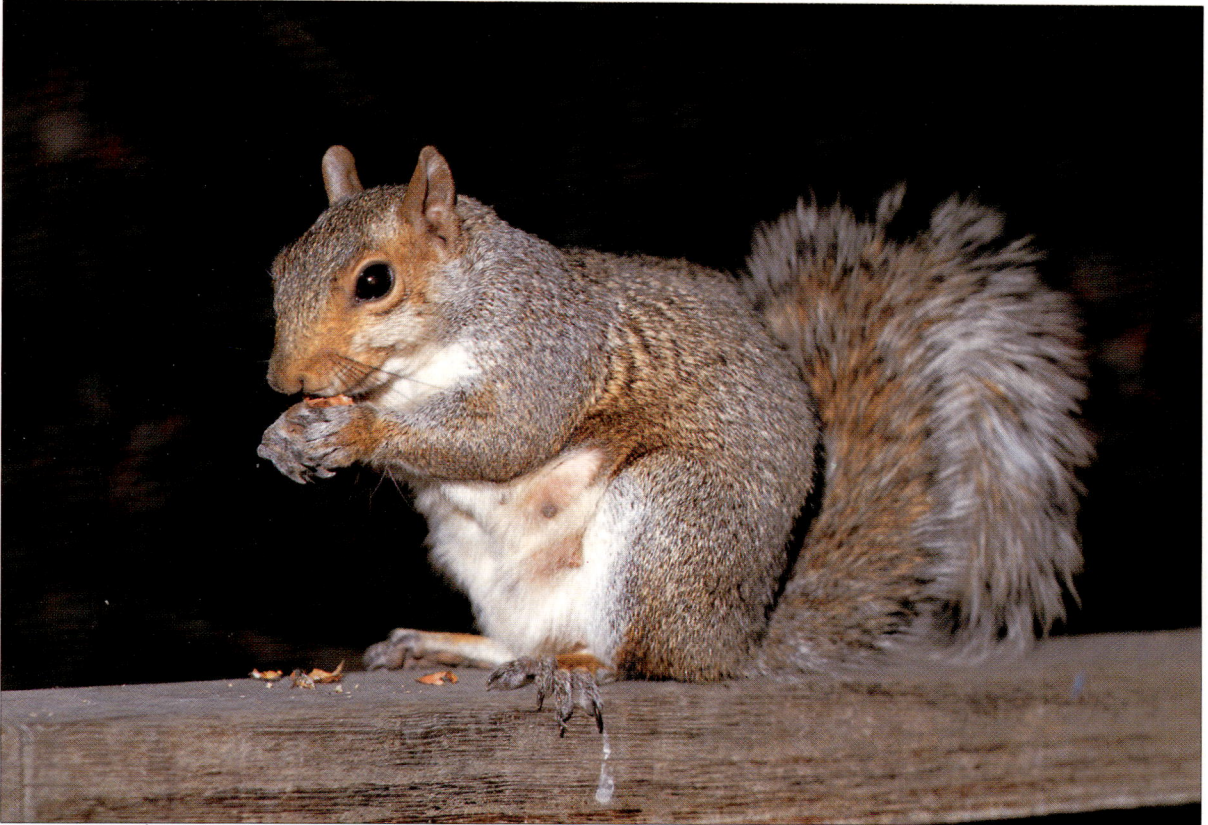

Nearly everything you eat contains some protein! Plants make protein from three things: water, **carbon dioxide** and **nitrogen**. The last two are gases found in the air. All animals get their protein either by eating plants or by eating other animals. Table 2 on page 18 shows the weight of protein in each 100 g of food.

*ABOVE* This squirrel is dining on a nut, which contains protein. All animals get their protein either by eating plants or other animals.

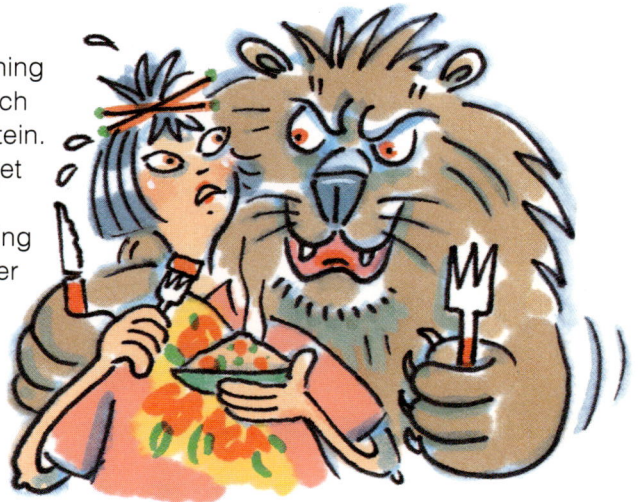

## Table 2

### Weight of protein in 100 g of some foods

| | Weight/100gm | | Weight/100gm |
|---|---|---|---|
| Milk | 3.3 | Peas | 5.0 |
| Yoghurt | 3.6 | Parsnips | 1.7 |
| Cheese | 25.4 | Potatoes | 1.4 |
| Bacon | 11.0 | Spinach | 2.7 |
| Beef | 14.8 | Apples | 0.3 |
| Chicken | 29.6 | Peanuts | 28.1 |
| Pork | 12.0 | Brown bread | 9.6 |
| Cod | 16.0 | White bread | 8.3 |
| Eggs | 11.9 | Barley, pearl | 7.7 |
| Butter | 0.5 | Brown rice | 2.5 |
| Baked beans | 6.0 | Soya flour | 52.0 |
| Broad beans | 7.2 | Wheat germ | 27.0 |

There are some surprises in this table. Some people think you have to eat lots of meat to get your protein. In fact this is not so. As you can see, soya flour actually contains more protein per 100 g than any of the meats on the list. Most vegetables also contain quite a lot of protein.

Soya beans come from a family of vegetables called pulses. All the peas and beans belong to this family, and they are wonderful foods. They give us large amounts of protein and can be grown all over the world. Grains are also useful for their protein. Look at the table and see how many different foods you can find that come from grains. How much protein would you get from 100 g of each one?

BELOW Some of the fish we buy has been farmed in special fish farms, where they have been fed and cared for at great cost.

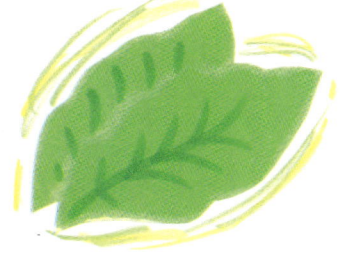

# Growing protein

Some of the foods on the list on page 18 come from plants and some from animals. Most of the meats on the list contain more protein than most of the plants. But animals that are kept for their meat have to be fed all through their lives, and the food they eat has to be grown. It takes much more farm land to produce meat than to grow vegetables, because the cows, pigs, sheep and other animals that we kill for their meat need lots of grass and grain to feed them every day of their lives. Growing all this food for animals takes a great deal of land.

Every day there are more people in the world, and we know that the number is sure to go on growing for many years. The world needs to produce more food to keep all those people alive. To do this, farm land needs to be used in the best way so that each hectare grows food for as many people as possible. By using farm land like this, we will help to keep some land wild for the animals and plants that have always lived there.

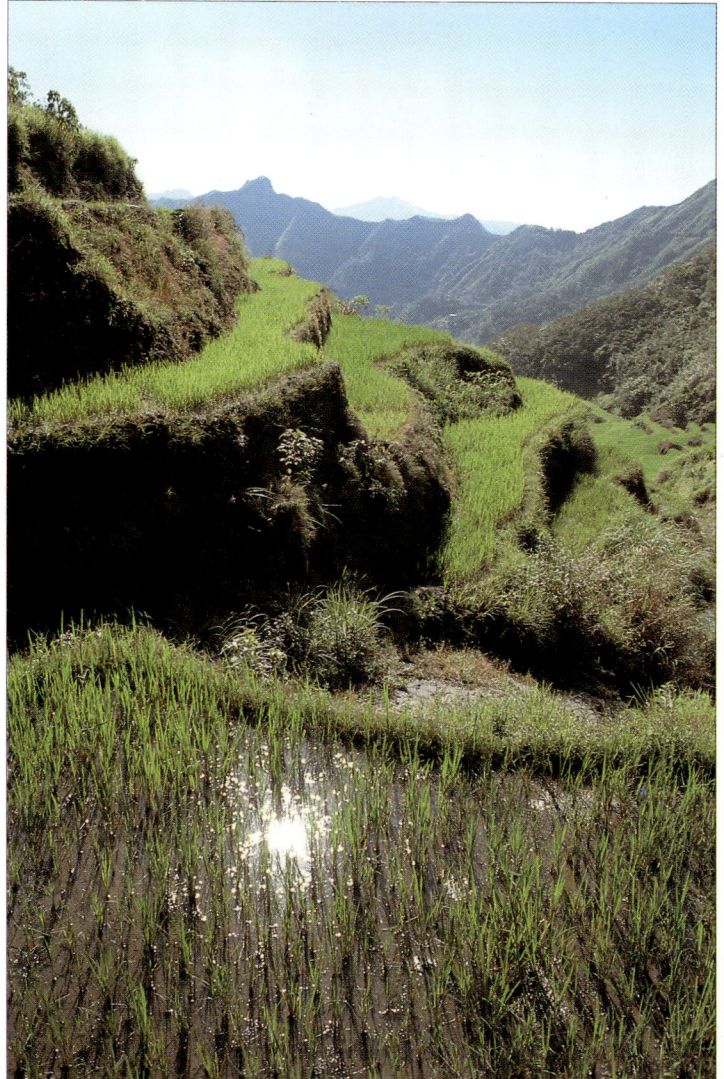

Often large areas of wild land are taken by farmers who need food for themselves and their animals, or crops to sell to earn money.

*ABOVE* Rice fields use farm land well, producing large amounts of food on a small area of land.

**Table 3**

| Table showing how much protein we get from different foods grown on 1 hectare of land | Kg of food per hectare | Kg of protein per hectare |
|---|---|---|
| Cereals | 875 | 87 |
| Pulses | 625 | 150 |
| Meat | 50 | 10 |
| Leafy vegetables | 12,500-25,000 | 500 – 10,000 |
| Root vegetables | 12,500-25,000 | 250 – 600 |
| Fruit | 25,000-50,000 | 200 – 400 |

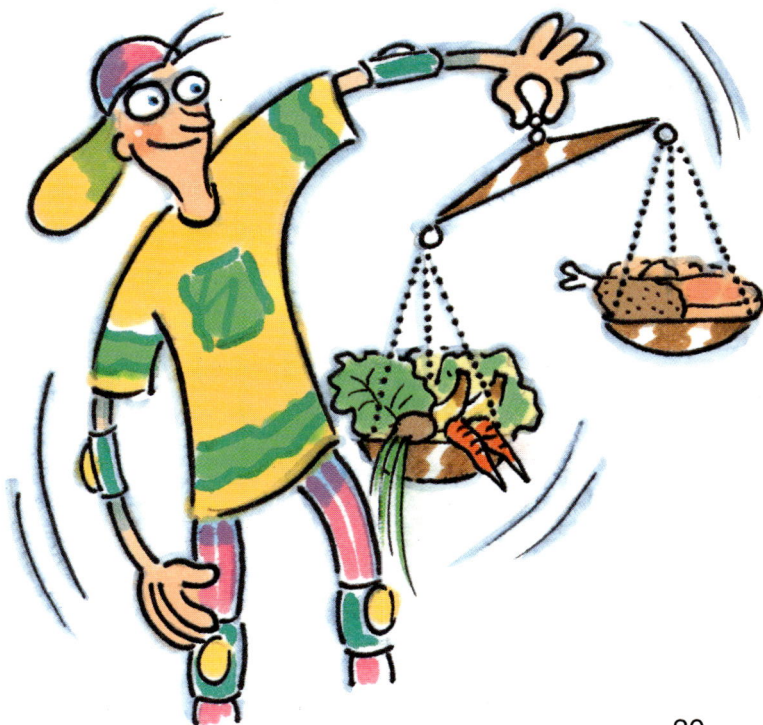

Table 3 shows different kinds of foods. For each kind, you can see how many kilogrammes of food are produced per hectare of land (column 1) and how many kilogrammes of protein we get from food grown on one hectare (column 2).

The information in this chart is quite startling. It shows very clearly how wasteful it is to use a lot of farmland in a crowded world just to rear animals for food. Some of this land could give us very much more protein (as well as all the other nutrients we need) if we used it to grow plants. In fact a meat-free diet could be a good answer to feeding the hungry people in the world today. Some people believe it may be the only way to feed the extra millions of people we expect the world to contain, until we manage to stop the human population from getting any bigger.

*BELOW* This meal of chicken with vegetables is well balanced. It contains a good mix of all the vital nutrients. However, it is also quite possible to have well-balanced meals that do not contain any meat at all.

However, the table does not tell us anything about the kind of protein in each food. To get the right mixture for our bodies to grow strong and healthy, we need to eat food from different groups. We must make sure that we eat a variety of foods, which, when put together, give us a balanced diet. We can do this by eating both meat and plants, or by eating many different kinds of food plants.

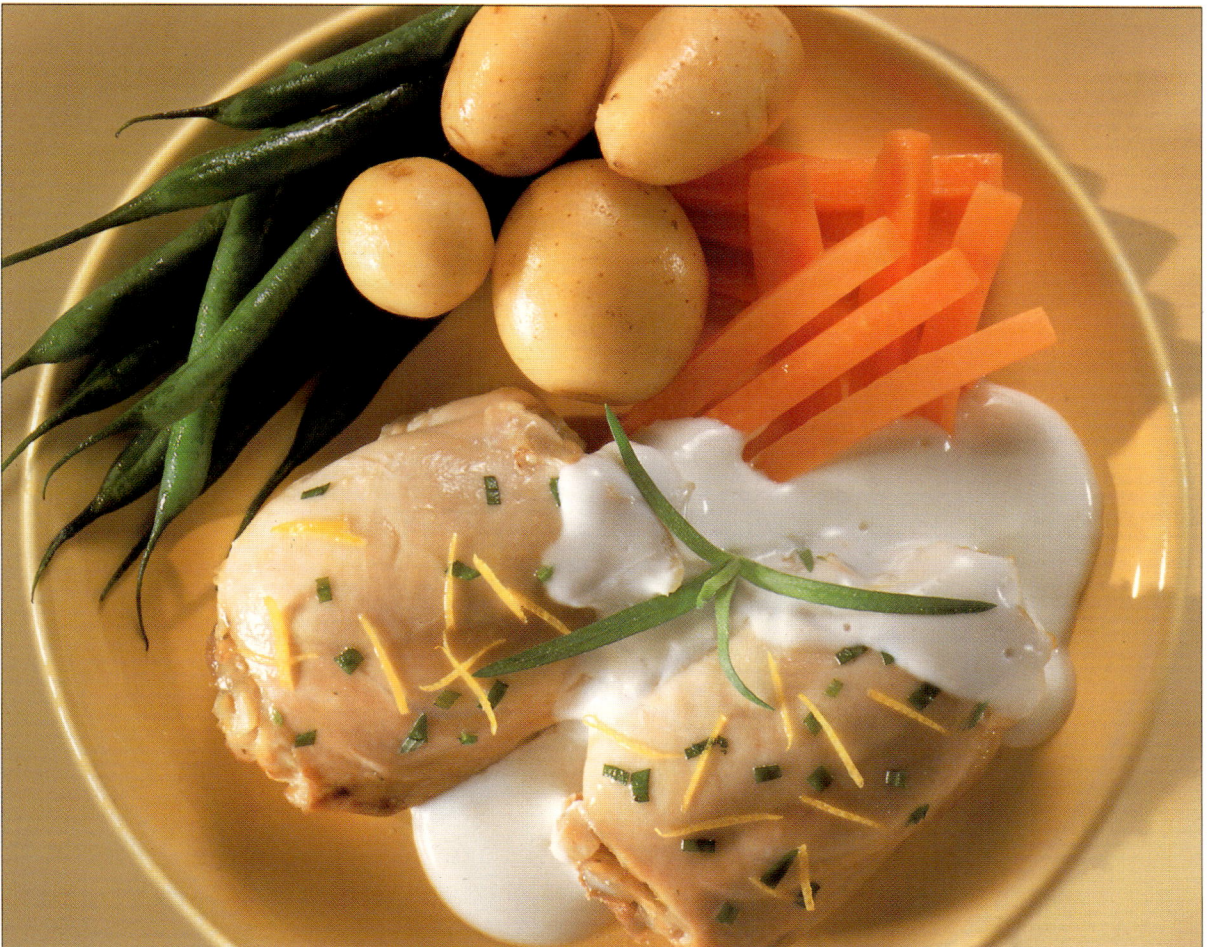

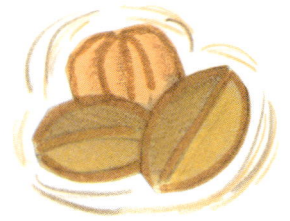

# How the world eats

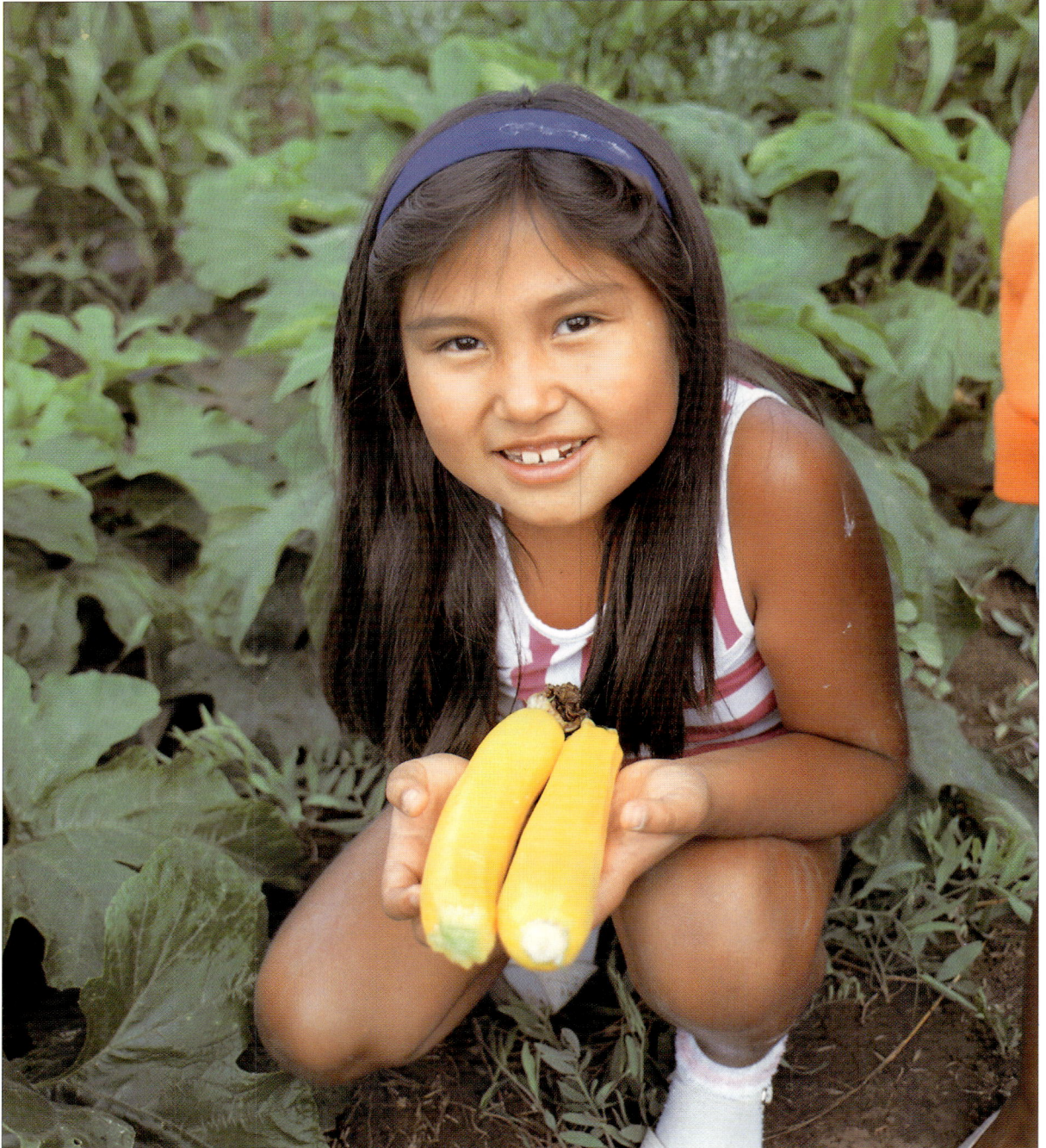

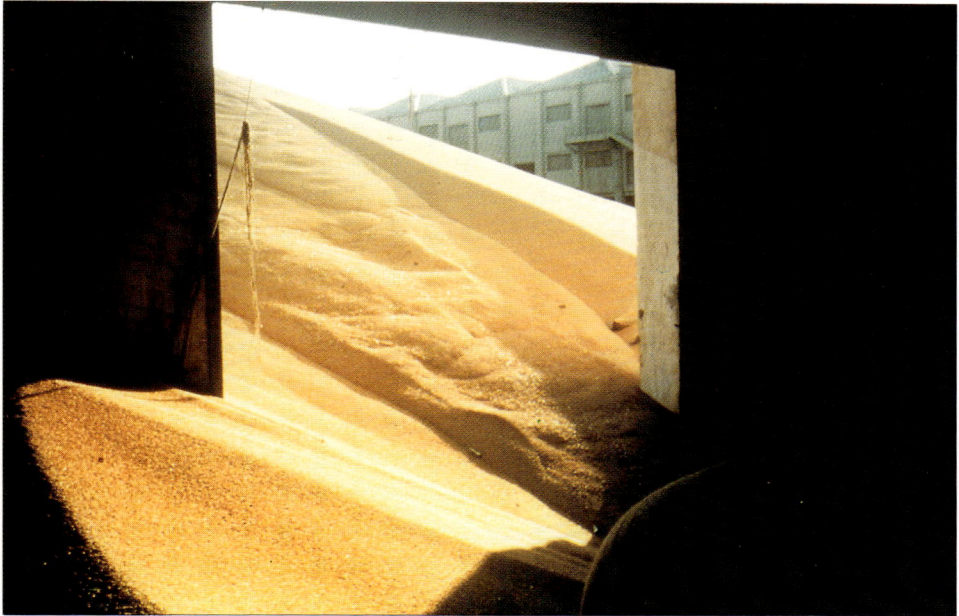

*RIGHT* This grain store in a Western country is bursting with extra grain, whilst many people in the world are starving to death. Lack of food is not always the problem. For many countries the problem is how to pay for it.

*OPPOSITE* To grow a healthy crop like these marrows, fertile soil, sunshine and plenty of rain are necessary. When there is not enough rain, the crop shrivels up and dies.

If we look around the world we will find people have very different ways of eating. Rich countries like Britain and the USA eat many different kinds of foods from all over the world. Most people have enough to eat, and some of us eat too much. Many of us eat an unhealthy diet, with too much sugar and fat. We may also eat more protein than we need.

You have probably seen pictures on your television of people dying of hunger when a really bad **famine** is in the news. A famine happens when a country does not have enough rain to grow food, or cannot feed its people for some other reason, like war.

Then thousands of people starve to death and newspapers all over the world write about the disaster. We can see dreadful pictures on our televisions, and try to raise money to help.

But it is easy to forget that many people in poor countries are always hungry. They may not die of hunger, but they never have enough to eat. They can suffer from many diseases. Children who never get enough protein suffer from a disease called kwashiorkor. They have swollen stomachs and very little energy. Any slight illness may kill them as they have not enough strength to fight it off.

# Where to get your protein

If you eat meat, quite small helpings each day will give you enough protein. Try not to eat too much meat; remember a lot of meat is not good for your body and is not good for your planet!

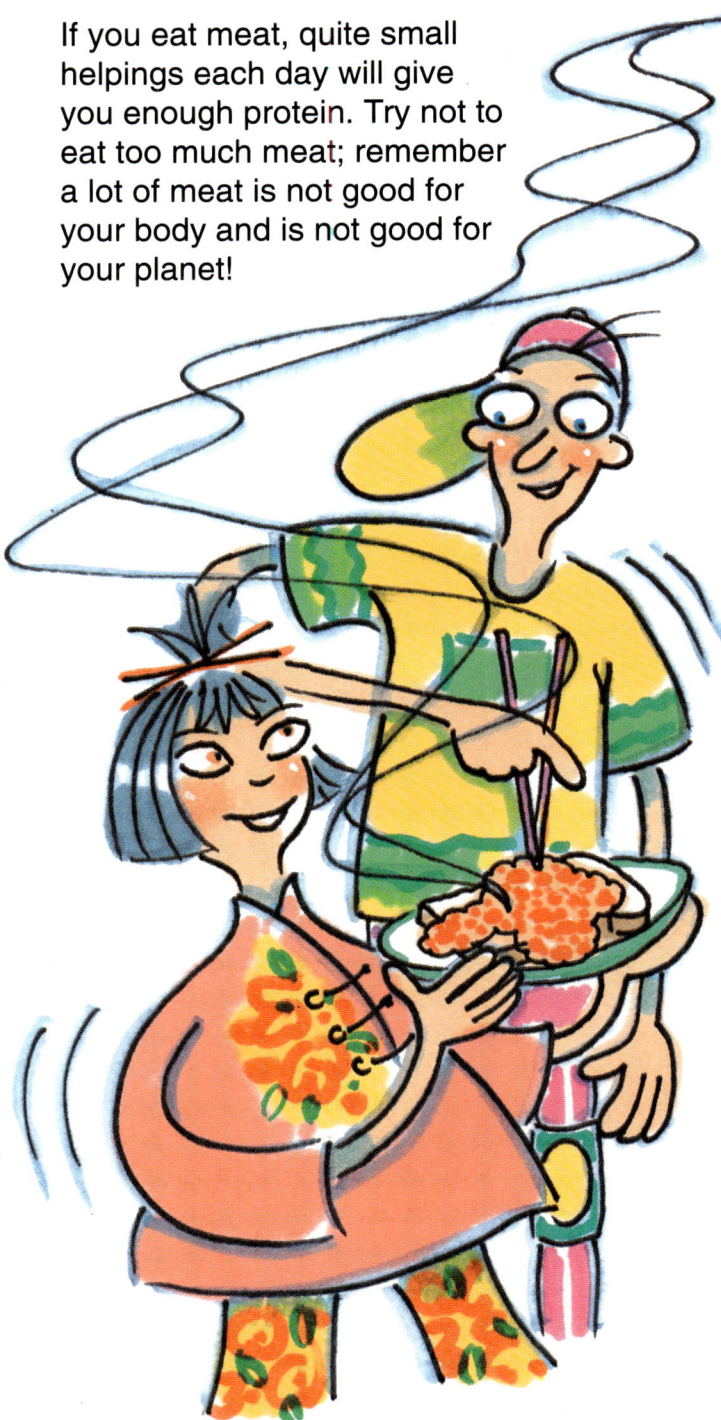

Cheese, milk and eggs, which are also animal food products, are also rich in protein and you do not need very much of them to get enough for your daily needs. However, many people believe that the main hope for feeding our planet's growing number of people lies in using more plant foods. You can learn to do this at home, and discover all sorts of delicious recipes at the same time!

Some of them will not be new to you. Baked beans on toast is a common meal for most of us, and it's a very good example of protein combining. This means using two kinds of protein at the same time to get a better quality protein.

On the whole, foods that come from animals give us higher quality protein, with more EAAs, than foods that come from plants. Some groups of plant foods do not have one EAA, some are short of another. But if we put foods from different groups together, we get much better quality protein than if we eat the same

24

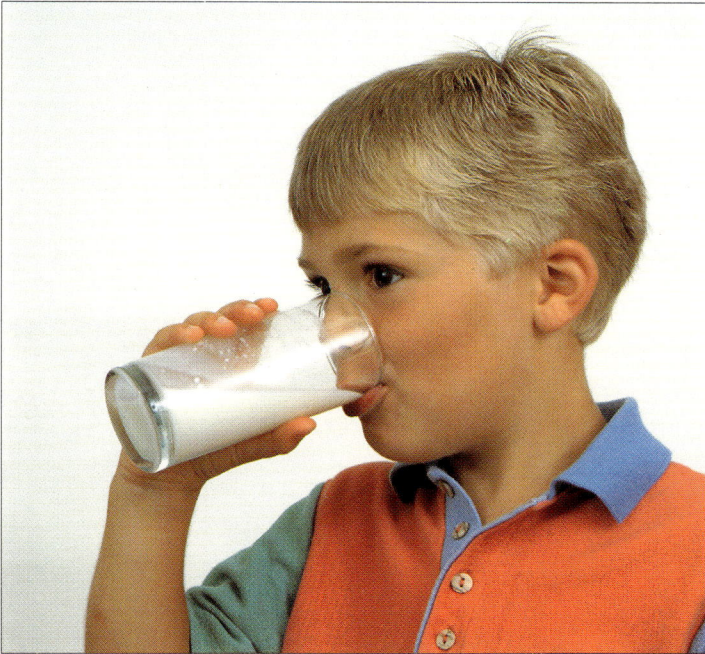

LEFT
A glass of milk is rich in protein and vitamins, but it also contains a lot of fat.

BELOW
This colourful assortment of grains and pulses is packed with protein.

These combinations give good quality protein and can be used instead of meat, or to replace some of the meat or fish you eat.

Quite small amounts of meat or fish will give you all the protein you need, and if you eat more foods from the other groups, you will need even less animal protein.

amount of the two foods separately.

Here are some groups of protein foods that come from animals: meat, fish, eggs, milk, and milk products (cheese and yoghurt). Protein-giving foods that come from plants include grains, pulses, seeds and nuts.

Why not try to increase the number of different protein groups in your diet? The best way to do this is to learn to combine groups of plant proteins. Here are some examples:

*pulses with grains*
*grains with nuts or seeds*
*nuts or seeds with pulses*

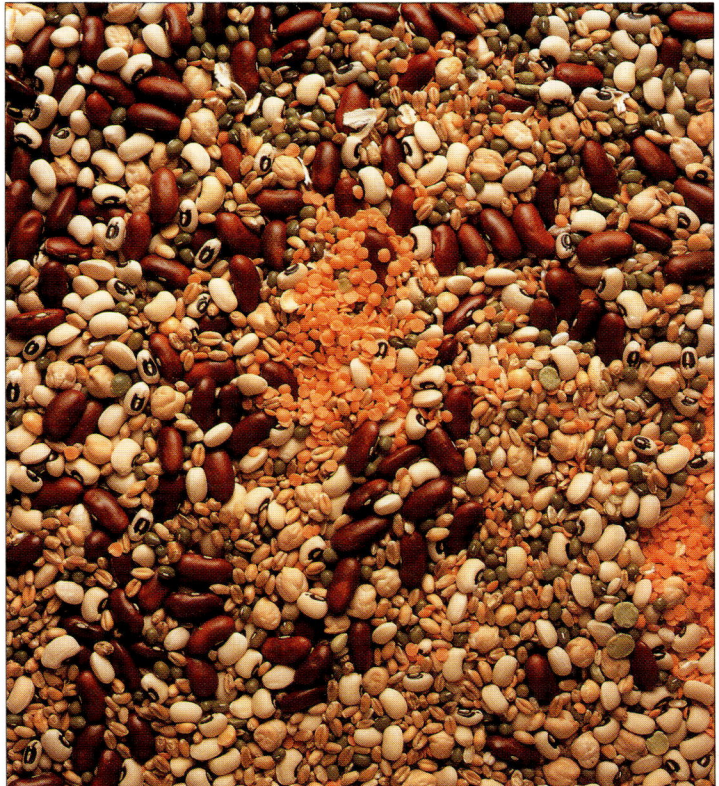

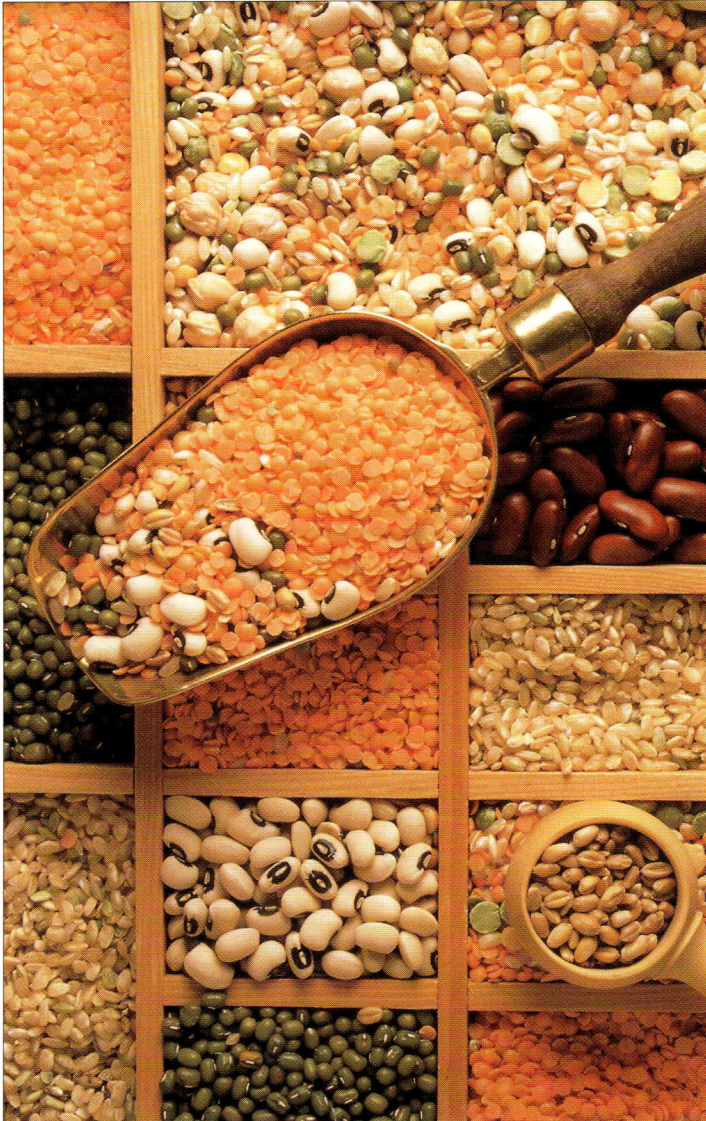

1.1 litres of water to each 450 g of wheat. Ask an adult to help you to bring the water to the boil in a large pan, add the wheat, reduce the heat and simmer with a lid on for 1½ hours or as long as it takes to soften the grains. They won't get really soft like cooked rice, but feel crunchy. Add a little salt when cooked.

*Bulgar wheat.* Although common in many parts of the world, this useful grain is not well known in Britain. It is partly prepared when you buy it. The grain has been cooked in water, dried and cracked before being packed. So it doesn't take long to cook. The easiest way to prepare it is to pour 450 ml of boiling water on to 225 g of bulgar wheat in a large bowl and simply leave it to swell and soften. Ask for help with the boiling water.

*Pulses.* You can buy most of the dried beans and peas in this family already cooked in tins. They are cheap and quick to use, so it's a good idea to have some in the food cupboard. But it's even cheaper, and quite easy, to grow and cook them yourself. It just takes time!

*ABOVE* How many of these grains and pulses can you recognize?

## Some unusual foods to start with:

*Wholewheat grains.* These are delicious. Buy them in a wholefood shop and soak them in water for a few hours before cooking. To cook, use

## Sprouting your own seeds

When seeds sprout they become much richer in many nutrients, especially protein. You can grow your own sprouts at home easily and cheaply, and you can eat the sprouts raw or lightly cooked.

*You will need:*
A jam jar
A piece of muslin
Some seeds (alfalfa, chick peas, mung beans or soya beans)

*Method*
1. Soak 2 – 3 tablespoons of the seeds you have chosen in warm water overnight.
2. Rinse the seeds in cold water and drain them.
3. Put the seeds in the jar and cover the top with muslin.
4. Rinse in cold water once or twice a day until the sprouts are long enough to eat (this takes 3 – 5 days).
5. Rinse, drain and serve.

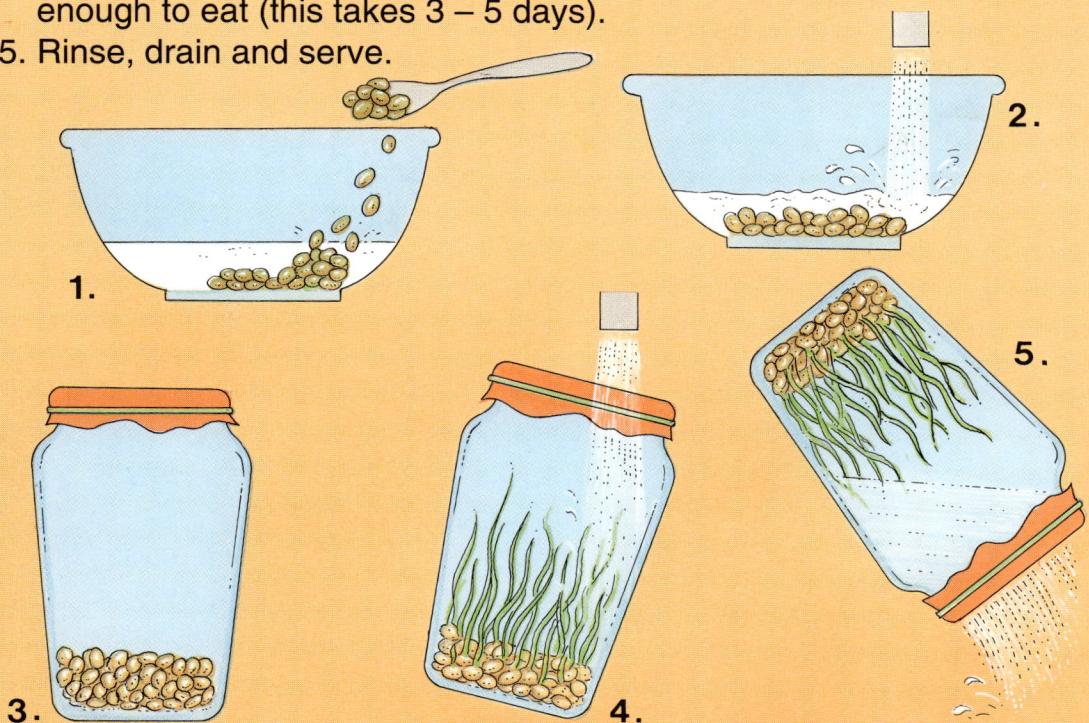

# Your daily protein

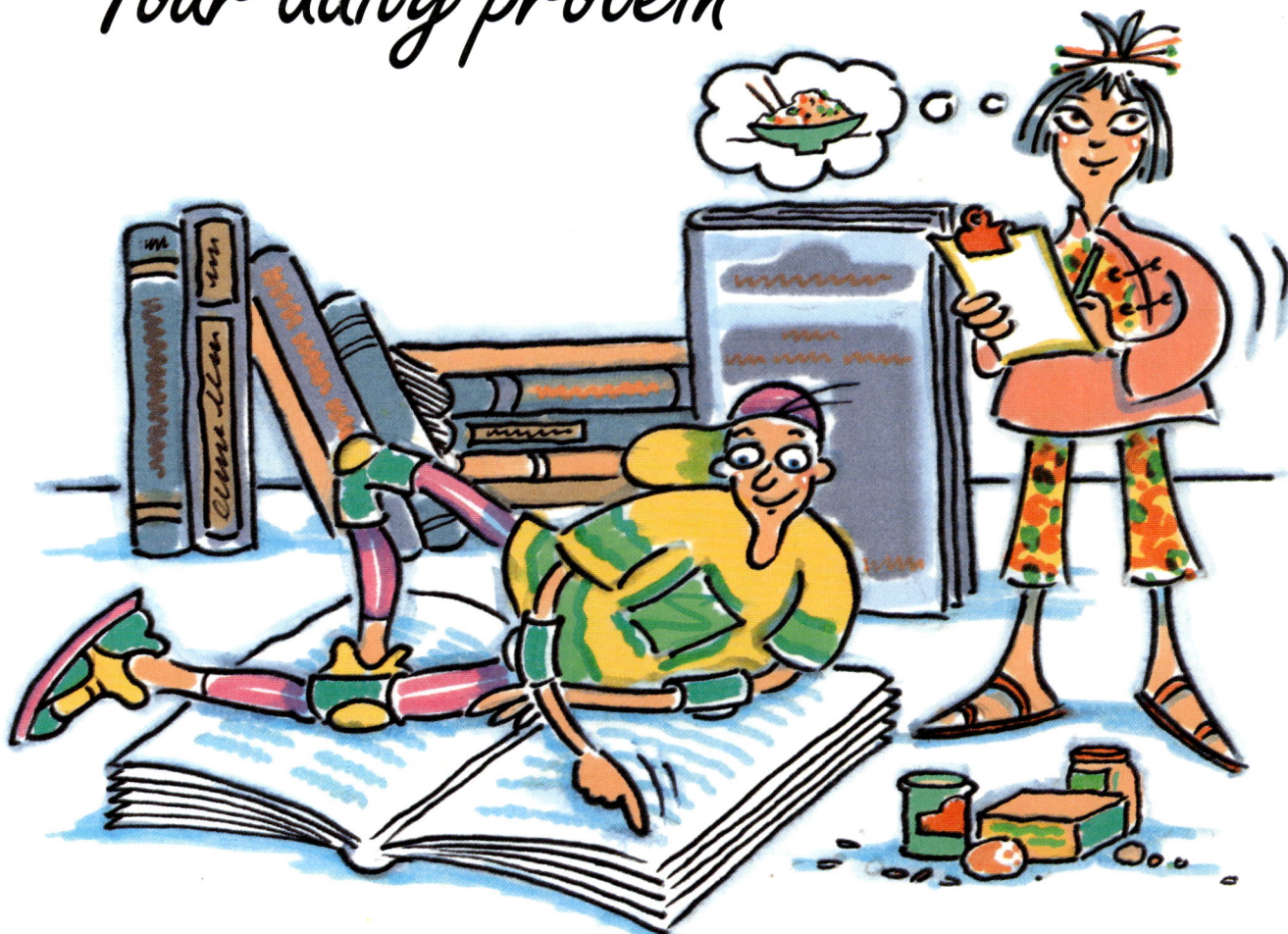

Try to find out how much protein you're eating and where it comes from. You will need to keep a note of everything you eat on one day. When you have chosen the day, plan ahead. You'll need a notebook and scales to weigh your food, and help from whoever cooks it. Packets and tins can be very helpful. Most of them tell you on the label how much protein (and other things) there is in 100 g. You can use the table on page 18 to help you find out this kind of information too. Perhaps you can use your school library or the public library to find a book with more facts about protein in food.

Write down how much you have eaten of all the different foods that make up the day's meals. Then try to find out how much protein there is in 100 g of each food. Now you can do a sum for each food and work out how many grammes of protein you have eaten. How does it compare with the amount in the table on page 15? Does most of your protein come from animals? How much comes from plants? Did any of your meals combine protein foods from the different groups on page 25?

Opposite is a list of meals that combine different proteins. Some of them you'll know. Some may sound strange at first. But they are well worth trying out, and you can add more of your own. Why not make a recipe book of good meals using different mixtures of protein?

Once you start finding out about what's in your food, and thinking about eating in a healthy way (good for you, and good for your planet), you will have a new interest which can last all through your life. We all need to eat every day, and we all have some choice about what we eat. As you get older you'll have even more choice, and you'll be able to join in more and more with shopping and cooking. Good luck with the food of the future!

Protein-packed meals

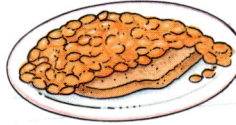

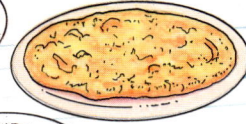

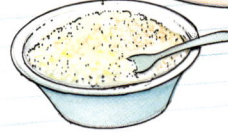

Beans on toast.

Porridge with milk.

Muesli with milk.

Rissoto with minced beef or chicken.

Rice pudding.

Cauliflower cheese with brown breadcrumbs or ground nuts.

Pasta salad with tuna.

Pizza with grated cheese.

Brown rice salad with mixed beans.

Spicy bulgar wheat salad with pine nuts.

Cooked wheat grains with mixed vegetables (hot or cold).

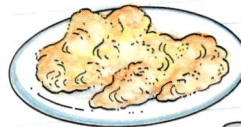

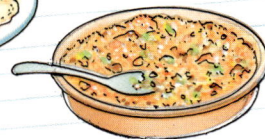

# Glossary

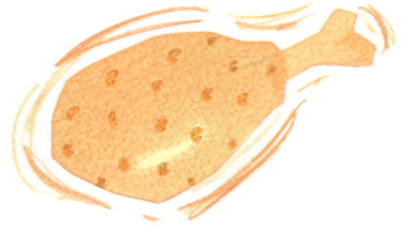

**Amino acids**   Parts of a protein.

**Architect**   Someone who designs buildings.

**Carbon dioxide**   One of several gases in the air we breathe.

**Cell**   A tiny part of a living thing, which cannot be seen with the naked eye.

**Convert**   Change into.

**Expert**   Someone who has made a special study of a subject.

**Famine**   A shortage of food.

**Nitrogen**   A gas which forms nearly 80 per cent of the air we breathe.

**Nutrients**   The things our bodies need from food to remain fit and healthy.

**Population**   The number of people living somewhere.

# Books to Read

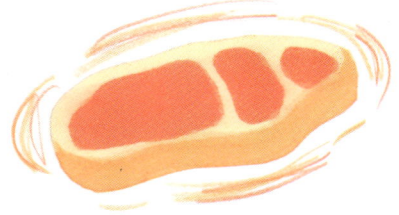

*Captain Eco and the Fate of the Earth*, Jonathan Porritt and Ellis Nadler (Dorling Kindersley, 1991)

*Famine in Africa*, Lloyd Timberlake (Franklin Watts, 1990)

*Burgers and Bugs: The Science Behind Food*, Lesley Newson (Piccolo, 1991)

*Diet*, Brian Ward (Franklin Watts, 1991)

*Beans*, Terry Jennings (A & C Black, 1991)

*Some People Don't Eat Meat*, Jane Inglis (Oakroyd Press, 1991)

## Picture Acknowledgements

Chapel Studios 25; Bruce Coleman 8, 19, 22; Ecoscene 9; Eye Ubiquitous 11; Chris Fairclough 5,14, 17; Science Photo Library 21, (bottom), 26; Wayland Picture Library 6, 12,23; Zefa 7, 10, 12,18.

# Index

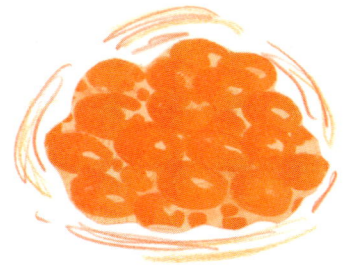